Walking Down The Path

To Multiple Sclerosis

One woman's
personal battle with
Primary Progressive Multiple Sclerosis

Sheril Lee

ACKNOWLEGEMENTS

Many thanks to T.J.O. for helping me edit this book, and T. and C. for urging me to tell my story.

PLEASE NOTE
This book does not provide medical advice. Should you want or need medical help or guidance, please consult your health care provider or physician.

TABLE OF CONTENTS

Prologue

This book is a true story based on the life of a woman who has battled Multiple Sclerosis for over thirty years. It is also about the fore-warnings she was given concerning her future with MS, and what would happen to her down the road. Did this insight come from God? Did it come from the universe or a higher power? She does not know. All she knows is that she benefited by paying attention to these premonitions.

You might notice the print in this book is a larger size. It has a 14 point size font. Many books and websites use a smaller 8 point or 10 point size font. The larger size print is to make it easier for anyone who has limited vision to enjoy the book. To appreciate the size difference here is an example of an 8 point size, and a 10 point size.

CHAPTER 1

I was born and raised in Indiana. My mom and dad had three daughters. I was the middle child. My older sister and my little sister were both quiet, reserved children. Then there was me, loud and full of energy. My father called me wiggle butt because I could not sit still. He would sit on a chair and I would climb onto his lap. I would lay my head on his chest and snuggle close to him. Then without warning, I would suddenly raise my head and smack him on the chin. He ended up with two chipped teeth because of me.

My first experience with the unusual happened when I was two years old. My older sister and I were sitting on the floor. We were rolling a ball between our legs when all of a sudden I turned blue and fell backward onto the floor. Panicked, my mother rushed me to the hospital. Mom must have been doubly scared that day because years ago when she was a young girl, her little sister died at the age of two from meningitis. I was named after my mother's sister. She died when she was two, and I was two when this happened. Luckily I survived. The doctors had no idea why I turned blue and stopped breathing. Why did I survive? God must have had a reason for me to live and to return home to my family.

When I was 12, I fell down and sprained my right wrist. Being right handed, the sprain made it hard for me to write. My parents weren't happy with me when I tried writing with my left hand. At first my writing was horrible, but eventually, it became readable. When my wrist was okay, I continued to alternate between my left hand and my right hand. My goal was to be ambidextrous.

Throughout my life, I switched hands regularly. I bowled right handed, but occasionally I would bowl with my left hand. I dealt cards left-handed, much to the teasing of my younger sister. When I would leap over a puddle, I would push off with my left leg. That's something a right handed person usually wouldn't do. They would use their right leg to push off.

When I was diagnosed with Multiple Sclerosis, my right side became my weaker side. Even today my left side is stronger than my right. My left leg and my left arm are currently used as if I had been left handed all my life. There is one exception. I'm still able to write with my right hand, even though my vision problems have slowed me down. Was it difficult becoming left handed? No. After all, I had been switching between my right hand and my left hand for years. I believe God slowly prepared me for the day MS would change my life.

My first job out of High School was with an airline. I was a Reservationist for Ozark Airlines. My job was to book seats on Ozark, and other airlines, for those passengers who called on the telephone.

While working for Ozark Airlines, I experienced my first feeling of being guided along. There was something deep down inside me that was pushing me to travel, and travel I did. I found the urge to fly ironic because I was a white-knuckle flier. That means I had a fear of flying. When the airplane prepared to take off or land, I gripped the armrests so tightly my knuckles would turn white. Even though I was apprehensive about flying, I traveled as often as my finances allowed.

Although I received free or reduced air travel on Ozark Airlines and discounted airfare on the other airlines, I needed money to pay for hotels and sightseeing. When I left Indiana, my parents gave me a mixed bag of items like non-matching drinking glasses and silverware. Slowly I added more glasses to the few I had by going to any gas station that was giving away a drinking glass with an eight gallon fill up. To save money I bought TV dinners when they were on sale and ate more macaroni and cheese than I care to remember.

Periodically during the year, other airlines would throw a party for Ozark employees. The host airline would have a drawing for free airline tickets. The tickets were always to exciting destinations flown to by the host airline. One year I won a trip on Trans World Airlines (TWA). It was a trip around the world for two. How could I pass that up? A fellow co-worker and I traveled on TWA to Heidelberg, Germany; Lucerne, Switzerland; Athens, Greece; Bangkok, Thailand; Hong Kong; and Honolulu, Hawaii. I'm so glad my friend and I were able to have this great experience together. It was a trip of a lifetime!

The next thing that happened to me that made me think something else was guiding my life was a car accident. I was on my way home to see my folks. On a two-lane road outside the small town of Remington, Indiana I rolled my Volkswagen Beetle.

As I left the town, I found myself behind a slow moving truck. It was a big long semi-truck. I had driven this road many times, so I knew there was a long, straight stretch of road ahead. It had snowed that morning, and slush was flying off the side of the semi. The speed limit at that time was

70 mph, and the truck was going too slow for me. I dropped back a little and revved up the bug to a nice passing speed. When I got alongside the truck, I noticed a car down the road coming toward me. The following events happened in mere seconds, but a lot happened in that brief period.

When I saw the car coming toward me, I decided to drop back into my lane, back behind the truck. I tapped the brakes to slow down. The car started sliding. First it turned to the left, and I saw the left side of the road. Then the car turned to the right, and I faced the side of the semi truck. I could feel the car starting to be pulled toward the underside of the truck. I didn't want to hit the oncoming car head on, and I didn't want to be dragged under the truck. I thought *I'm going to die*, and wondered why my life wasn't flashing before my eyes. That is when I believe something outside of myself helped me think.

I began watching the telephone poles go by my left side window. When my car turned back toward the oncoming car, I saw a telephone pole go past me. At that same exact moment, I cranked the steering wheel all the way to the left and stood on the brakes. The next thing I remember was looking out my side window and seeing the ground, then the sky, and then the ground again. My Volkswagen Bug was rolling side over side.

When the car stopped rolling it was laying on its side. The passenger side of the car was down on the ground, and the driver's side was up where the roof should have been. I was half dangling in the air because the seat belt I was wearing was holding me fast to my seat. The radio was blasting and a small hard sided makeup case, that had been in the backseat, was now in the front passenger seat. I remember feeling the suitcase brush past my head when the car was rolling over. I had no idea it had flown past me from the backseat to the front seat, smashing into and cracking the front window.

I released my seat belt and fell onto the passenger window. When I turned off the radio, I could hear the car wheels still spinning and my turn signal clicking away. There was no way I could get out of the car through the doors, so I looked at the sunroof. It was to my right, where my passenger door should have been. I could not understand why it would not open more than a few inches. Why was it jammed? Frustrated I put my shoulder in the small opening and physically forced it open. Somehow I got the strength to move that crushed sunroof. When I crawled out the sunroof, I was looking at a telephone pole approximately 14 inches away from my face.

Why did my car start to slide? What went wrong? Later I learned that I had passed from one county into another one right after I started to pass the truck. The first part of the road had been salted. When I was beside the truck, I passed from one county into the next one. That part of the road had not been salted. It was pure ice. In the next two hours four other vehicles went off the road into the ditches, on the same stretch of road. Two of them resulted in deaths.

Why was I spared? I walked away from an accident with little more than glass in my hair, and days later, muscle spasms all up and down my back.

It was never easy to travel that same stretch of road again. Later that year, as I traveled home over the Thanksgiving weekend, a warning light in my Volkswagen Beetle came on. Guess what city I was near? Remington, Indiana. The small city, with a population of approximately 1,200 people, was not done with me. The alternator brushes had burned out. At least that is what the owner of the small gas station told me. Eventually, the brushes were replaced, and I continued on my way home.

My car accident was the first of several traumatic events that happened that year. My father suffered a heart attack, my mother had cancer surgery and my parent's garage went up in flames. As awful as those events were, none of them could compare to our family's greatest tragedy. My older sister was killed in a car accident. The way she died was eerily similar to my car accident. The car she was riding in had an electrical failure. The headlights went out as the car was going around a curve on a dark, two-lane country road. The car ran off the road and hit a telephone pole. My sister was killed instantly. She was 24 years old. She left behind 2 loving parents, 2 loving sisters, and 1 loving husband.

My sister's accident also left me wondering why she had died and I hadn't. Her death scared me. Would I die young as she had? Would I die when I was 24? It was then that I decided to speed up everything in my life. If it meant I used up every penny I had, I was going to go everywhere and do everything as fast as I could. I was bound and determined to see as much of the world as possible.

CHAPTER 2

A year later I took my next trip. The most exotic and thrilling place I could think of was Nairobi, Africa. Traveling with my parents, we toured several national parks. The first night in Africa we stayed at the Mount Kenya Safari Club. Each room had a mosquito net over the bed and a real wood burning fireplace. Our first night's dinner consisted of a buffet of exotic meats and fruits. Where else could I try lion, antelope, zebra, or ostrich meat? The Safari Club had its own animal preserve. One special memory I will remember forever was the day I went horseback riding around their preserve. I got to see small herds of antelope, giraffes, zebra, and elephants close up.

When we left the Mt. Kenya Safari Club we headed out on a safari tour of the Tsavo National Park. We traveled in a touring van with an open sunroof. We were joined by a father who was traveling with his 27-year-old daughter. If anyone of us saw something we wanted to photograph, the driver would stop and we would stand up and take the shot out of the sunroof.

Our driver drove around looking for herds of animals. On the dirt road, or off the road and through the brush he would drive, trying to find animals for us to see and photograph. It was exciting when he spotted a pride of lions lying in the shade of some dry bushes. The lions were not scared off by the van, so the driver was able to get within 60 feet of them. It was a photographers dream.

Next, we headed to the Tree Top Lodge. This hotel was unusual because it was elevated above the ground. The lodge was built next to a watering hole. From the veranda, visitors could quietly watch the animals come to drink at the watering hole. To see certain nocturnal animals, a member of the staff would come to your room at night, and tell you to hurry to the viewing area. The animals were so close I could have thrown a tennis ball and hit them. It was an extraordinary way to see free roaming animals.

Several years later I left Ozark Airlines and started working as a Sales Representative for Swissair. Swissair is the national airline of Switzerland. One of my jobs was to make travel arrangements for various groups traveling on

Swissair. The job required that I personally see the groups off at the airport, and at a later date greet them at the airport upon their return home. Most of the groups flew out of New York. I would fly with the group from Chicago to New York to make sure everything went smoothly, and everyone got on their Swissair flight to Europe. When the group returned, I would fly to New York to greet them and welcome them back to the United States. Then we would all fly to Chicago together. Believe me, all of this flying back and forth caused me to have a lot of anxiety and white-knuckles!

One trip, in particular, stands out in my mind. Swissair asked me to be a tour coordinator for a group of travel agents. My job was to make sure the group stayed together and everything went smoothly. Whether boarding an airplane or boarding a tour bus, my job was to make sure no one was left behind.

Our destination was Split, Yugoslavia. Once we arrived in Split, I turned everything over to the local tour guides. That left me free to sit back and enjoy the tour like everyone else. At one of our evening dinners, I bought wine for everyone compliments of Swissair. It was a wonderful trip. What made it extra special was the fact that Swissair picked up my tab for everything.

Three years later I left Swissair and started to work for Federal Express. Federal Express (now FedEx) is a cargo airline. If you think my days of flying were over, you would be wrong. Federal Express had reciprocal agreements with the other airlines. That allowed me to travel at reduced rates on most passenger airlines.

Occasionally I had to fly to Memphis, Tennessee for company training. To get to

Memphis, I would fly on a Federal Express jet. I would sit in the jump seat, which is a small seat located inside the flight cabin, right behind the pilot. Talk about a front row seat! I could see and hear everything that was going on the cockpit.

The scariest flight I ever took was on a Federal Express Falcon 20 Jet. We were returning home from Memphis. Due to a bad snowstorm, we were unable to land. We circled the Chicago airport as the ground crew worked to clear the snow off the runways. In the cockpit I was wearing headphones that allowed me to listen to the communications between all the pilots and the control tower. I heard my pilot tell the control tower that he only had 800 pounds of fuel left, and that he needed to land now.

The wind was blowing our plane sideways as we started to land. I was scared and holding on for dear life. The snow had been cleared off the runway, but there were many icy patches here and there. We did a little sliding, but luckily we landed safely. Inside the terminal I asked the pilot what he meant when he told the control tower we only had 800 pounds of fuel. He told me we had 10 minutes of fuel left. We HAD to land. Glad I didn't know that when we were in the air. I would have been petrified with fear.

Several years later I had major dental work done. My teeth were in bad shape. I needed fillings in half of my teeth. Back then fillings contained Mercury. I find it suspect that three years later, after getting a mouth full of fillings, I experienced my first Multiple Sclerosis symptom. Did the fillings have anything to do with my MS? I don't know. There are anecdotal stories of people with MS having their fillings removed and returning to full health. All their signs of MS were gone. Wish I could have had my fillings removed.

Unfortunately, there were so many of them it wouldn't have been practical. I will never know if removing the fillings would have helped me.

CHAPTER 3

My first symptom of MS appeared soon after I was married. It all started with a little vision loss in my left eye. It was like I had a piece of thin plastic over my eye. A co-worker gave me the name of her Ophthalmologist. The next day I made an appointment. The doctor thought I had a mild infection and told me to come back in six weeks. On my second visit, the first doctor wasn't available, so I saw a different Ophthalmologist. He told me that I had a 5% to 10 % vision loss, but he didn't know why. He suggested I return in six weeks. He also suggested I see a Neurologist.

My vision had been 20/20 the last time I had a vision test, so although a 10% vision loss wasn't a lot, it bothered me. At work the blurriness was affecting my performance. It was hard to read forms and paperwork because my eyes couldn't focus on the print. I ended up tying a scarf over my left eye so I could look at paperwork with my good eye.

When I made an appointment to see a Neurologist he told me he thought I was nervous and scheduled an appointment for a VER-EEG.

Here's a quick explanation of a VER - *"Visual evoked response (VER) test. This test can diagnose problems with the optic nerves that affect sight. A healthcare professional places electrodes along your scalp to record the electrical signals as you watch a checkerboard pattern flash for several minutes on a screen."[1]*

[1] John Hopkins Medicine Health Library www.hopkinsmedicine.org http://www.hopkinsmedicine.org/healthlibrary/test_procedures/neurol ogical/evoked_potentials_studies_92,p07658/ accessed 06/26/2017

Here's a quick explanation of an EEG - *"An EEG is a test that detects abnormalities in your brain waves, or in the electrical activity of your brain. During the procedure, electrodes consisting of small metal discs with thin wires are pasted onto your scalp. The electrodes detect tiny electrical charges that result from the activity of your brain cells. The charges are amplified and appear as a graph on a computer screen, or as a recording that may be printed out on paper. Your healthcare provider then interprets the reading."[2]*

[2] John Hopkins Medicine Health Library www.hopkinsmedicine.org http://www.hopkinsmedicine.org/healthlibrary/test_procedures/ neurological/electroencephalogram_eeg_92,P07655/ accessed 06/26/2017

The EEG and VER test results came out okay

.

Four months after my first visit with an Ophthalmologist, I went to my family doctor. Told him about my blurriness and he gave me Valium and told me to come back in six weeks.

Now I was really frustrated. No one knew what was causing the blurriness in my eye and I was sick and tired of doctors telling me to come back in six weeks. Years later I decided that "come back in six weeks" really means "I have no idea what you have, but I'm hoping it will clear up and go away in six weeks!"

In the meantime, more upsetting symptoms were beginning to show up. I started experiencing dizziness, numbness, nervousness, and twitching. That is when I met Dr. Johnson. How lucky I was that he was filling in for my regular doctor that day. On our first visit I said to him in a prickly voice "If you're going to tell me I'm nervous and ask me to come back in six weeks, I might as well save us both time and leave now." From that moment on Dr. Johnson and I worked together to pinpoint my problem. He scheduled an EEG and an EKG. My Ophthalmologist had already sent me to have an EEG, but Dr. Johnson wanted his own test.

Here's a quick explanation of an EKG - *"An electrocardiogram (EKG or ECG) is a test that checks for problems with the electrical activity of your heart. An EKG shows the heart's electrical activity as line tracings on paper. The spikes and dips in the tracings are called waves."*[3]

[3] ByHealthwise Staff   webmd.com
Primary Medical Reviewer Rakesh K. Pai, MD, FACC - Cardiology, Electrophysiology
E. Gregory Thompson, MD - Internal Medicine

He also arranged for repeated glucose tests. Unfortunately, there was no clear-cut diagnosis.

Ten months after it started, the blurriness in my eye disappeared all by itself. I figured my eye problem was a fluke and I went on with my life.

The strong impulse I had to travel was still with me and urging me on. I continued to work for Federal Express and traveled as often as I could. My husband and I traveled to Lucerne, Switzerland; Vaduz, Liechtenstein; and Feldkirch, Austria.

Months later I woke up with numbness in my left hand and my left foot. The Orthopedic doctor had no idea why. He suggested I see a different Neurologist.

The new doctor could find no immediate reason for my numbness. She scheduled a BAER and a VER test. This would be my second VER test.

Here's a quick explanation of BAER - *"Auditory Brainstem Response Evaluations (ABR or BAER)   This test is non-invasive and is performed with recording electrodes placed on the forehead and ears. The audiologist will analyze recordings of electric potentials generated by the auditory neural pathway."* [4]

[4] John Hopkins Medicine
http://www.hopkinsmedicine.org/otolaryngology/specialty_areas/hearing/hearing-testing/abr.html
 accessed 6/26/2017

I had X-rays taken of my spine and more tests that would only bore you. She prescribed Zomax for the pain and set up vitamin B12 shots.

The shots made me sick, so I quit taking them. All the while the numbness continued.

After one year of no answers, I went to a Chiropractor. I was desperate to get rid of the numbness. I thought a Chiropractor might manipulate my numbness away. It's amazing what extremes a person will go to trying to get better.

CHAPTER 4

Four months later, while I was at work, I felt dizzy, and I experienced hot flashes. A co-worker drove me to the hospital where I was treated for hyperventilation. At this time I was feeling multiple symptoms that affected every part of my life. Besides the dizziness and hot flashes, I was suffering from numbness in my tongue, arms, legs, thighs, stomach, feet and hands. All over numbness scared me, but the numbness in my tongue really frightened me.

Immediately I made an appointment to see the neurologist. She set up a series of ACTH steroid shots for me.

Here's a quick explanation of ACTH - *"ACTH is a hormone made by the pituitary gland that tells the outer part of the adrenal gland to produce hormones such as cortisol. An ACTH stimulation test measures levels of cortisol in your blood before and after you are given a synthetic form of ACTH."*[5]

[5] Dartmouth-Hitchcock http://www.dartmouth-hitchcock.org/endo/acth.html#whatdoes accessed 06/26/2017

The shots were to be given twice a day for 21 days in a row. For 21 days I had to drive to the hospital to receive my shots. Every morning at 7:00 am I received a shot in my left hip. Every night at 7:00 pm I received a shot in my right hip.

Each shot was given in the same small quarter size area. Ouch! I felt like a pin cushion.

If you have ever taken steroids, especially over a long period of time, you know once you start you can't just stop. You have to be slowly weaned off of steroids. I was acutely aware of this.

One evening my husband drove me to the hospital. It was a terrifying drive for the both of us because we had to drive through a blinding snowstorm. The snowplows were clearing the freeways, but the main streets had not been plowed. As we drove past the back end of the airport, the wind had blown snow drifts across the two lane road. The streets were barely passable. Those of you who live in the northern states know a March snowstorm can be as big and brutal as a January storm. It was a long, nail-biting drive to the hospital. We were happy and relieved when we arrived safely and on time.

The steroids helped get rid of the majority of my numbness, but I still had it in my hands and feet.

It took a long time for the neurologist to give me her diagnosis. After more tests, the doctor finally told me I had Primary-Progressive Multiple Sclerosis (PPMS). During our previous visits the doctor had brought up the possibility of my having MS, but her diagnosis took me by surprise. It was official. I had Multiple Sclerosis.

What is PPMS? Unlike other forms of MS where a person has attacks followed by symptom-free periods, I was diagnosed with what I call a meaner kind of MS. PPMS patients experience a steady downward decline of their physical abilities. 1 out of 10 people with MS are diagnosed with PPMS. At the time I was diagnosed, there were no FDA-approved drugs for this type of MS.

The optimist in me refused to believe I had a disease that would never go away. I felt disappointed and let down because I knew MS could not be treated like a cold or the flu.

A month later I was desperate to stop the panic attacks I was experiencing. I started Biofeedback sessions.

Biofeedback was a way for me to learn how to relax and relieve some conditions I was experiencing. During my first biofeedback session, electrodes are attached to my skin and sensors were attached to my fingers. The electrodes and sensors sent signals to a monitor, which displayed an image that represented my heart rate, breathing rate, blood pressure, and skin temperature.

Through multiple sessions, I learned to control my breathing to reduce my stress level. The instructor told me to think the word *warm* as I learned how to control my breathing. The warmer my body became the worse I felt, so I began thinking the word *cool.* Fearing ridicule, I did not mention my new word to the instructor. Changing the word to cool helped a lot. Leave it to me to do things differently!

As if I didn't have enough troubles to deal with, I started to have panic attacks. If you have never had a panic attack, I will try to explain one to you, from my own personal experience. It is a sudden overwhelming rush of anxiety or fear that makes it hard for you to think logically. Anything can trigger an attack. You dread going out in public, and you fear leaving your house because you're afraid of losing control of yourself. Your heart starts to race, and you feel flushed. The more you think about losing control, the more hyper and out of control you become.

It becomes a vicious cycle that takes over your life and your anxiety begins to control you. Or should I say it takes over and stops your life?

Looking back, it is hard to imagine that this was one of my scary experiences. One sunny summer day I decided to walk to the end of the block and back. Unfortunately, I only made it three houses down before sheer panic kicked in. I was frozen in place. I remember looking down the street to the end of the block and then back at my house. My breathing became labored, my face felt hot, and I began to shake. All I wanted to do was turn around and run home as fast as I could. I didn't run, but I hurried home. It took weeks before I had the courage to walk halfway down the block.

Biofeedback helped control parts of my life that I felt were out of control. I will be forever grateful that it helped change my life for the better. By using Biofeedback, I was able to reduce my panic attacks without taking drugs. That was important to me.

Once the panic attacks were under control my husband, and I traveled to Paris, France. It was during this trip I experienced leg weakness and dizziness. Thankfully we were able to go to all the tourist spots even if I had to move more slowly than usual.

CHAPTER 4

After returning home from Paris my husband and I joined a dinner club that included six other couples. It was a fun group of co-workers and wives. We used to eat at different restaurants all around the city. The dinner club allowed everyone in our group to try foods we normally would not try. We would order multiple appetizers and pass them around for everyone to share. "May I try a bite" was often heard around the table. I always looked forward to these get-togethers.

One day the dinner club decided it would be a nice change of pace to go to a dog race track. One of the couples owned a large Recreational Vehicle and volunteered to drive us all to the track. That day, to my horror, I woke up with numbness all over my body including my face. There was numbness around my right eye, and down my right cheek. My tongue and lips were numb. The Multiple Sclerosis couldn't have flared up during a worse time.

My husband kept asking me if I was going to go. I desperately wanted to go, but I knew if I pushed too hard, what was now a temporary facial numbness might become permanent. Time was ticking down. Immediately I started using biofeedback to reduce my stress, and I prayed to God for help. Minutes before, and I really mean literally minutes before my husband was ready to leave, my tongue and lip numbness disappeared.

We joined the group, and off we went for a fabulous day at the race track - thanks to what I believe was some heavenly help.

One of the ladies in the dinner club had also been diagnosed with MS. We shared our stories and symptoms. Besides knowing each other through the dinner club, we both went to the same Neurologist.

My friend was diagnosed with relapsing-remitting MS. 65% to 80% of patients who have this type of MS experience a series of attacks followed by the complete or partial disappearance of the symptoms (known as remission) until another attack occurs (called a relapse). Many times there may be weeks to decades between relapses. There are several FDA-approved drugs for those who have relapsing-remitting MS.

Eight months had passed before I returned to see the Ophthalmologist. The blurriness in my right eye had returned. The doctor thought the problem was back in my Optic nerve. There was nothing he could do to help me. I was told to come back if the condition continued.

That May I mentioned to the Neurologist that I was having strong pains over my heart. It felt like someone was grabbing it and twisting it while applying pressure. This condition had been going on for six months. The doctor put me in the hospital to have my heart monitored. I stayed for five days while I had an ECHO M+2D that continuously monitored my heart. The diagnosis was Mitral Valve Prolapse, commonly called a floppy valve.

In addition to my floppy valve pain, the numbness was now all over my body, and I was having difficulty walking. All my health problems were being treated mainly by two doctors. They were in communication with each other, and they would pass me back and forth between them. Sometimes it felt like they were playing ping pong with me. First one, then the other would see me in their office and order tests.

The following week I went to see both doctors. One prescribed Inderol for my irregular heartbeat, and the other prescribed Dexamethasone (a steroid) for the numbness. While taking the steroids, I felt like I was given a preview of my future MS symptoms. By the end of June, most of the numbness was gone, except for the numbness in my hands and feet. Sadly the blurriness in my right eye remained.

Seven months later, in early December, I was thrilled when the blurriness disappeared. It completely disappeared! Two months later my husband and I took a trip to Hawaii with his three children. We had a wonderful time. We went everywhere and did everything tourists do in

Hawaii. It was a trip we will all remember forever.

My joy was short lived. Three short months later, after our return from Hawaii, things went downhill quickly. Both eyes became blurry. The eye doctor believed the problem was somewhere in my optic nerve.

That was when I felt a strong sense of urgency that NOW was the time to sell our two story condominium. Deep down inside I knew my MS was not going to go away. We needed to look for a ranch house where everything was on one level. It was getting harder for me to climb up and down the stairs. We put our condo up for sale.

It was hard for me to believe that in a few short years after I experienced my first MS symptom, the Ophthalmologist decided it was time for me to quit working. I could no longer read print or read the computer screen. There were no computer screen magnifiers available to help me at work, and eyeglasses only increased the blurriness.

He prescribed Decadron, another steroid. I had a bad, bad reaction to Decadron. While taking it, I lost the use of my legs and had difficulty breathing. There was tightness in my chest that felt like a vise around my ribs. For three days I lay in the fetal position on the living room floor. The pain was so great I could barely move. If I could have stopped taking the steroids, I would have in a heartbeat, but once you start taking steroids, you can't stop abruptly. I had to complete the ten-day course no matter how awful they made me feel. Once again steroids gave me a preview of what I could expect down the road with my MS. After no improvement in my condition, I went on Long Term Disability with Federal Express.

During those unsettling years, I kept a list of everything that had to do with my problem. The doctors' names and the dates I saw them. I made a list of the diagnostic tests and the steroids I had taken. The list was started because each new doctor wanted to know my medical history. I got tired of repeating everything over and over again. It was easier to hand them a piece of paper than verbally tell them. All in all, I went to see a Neurologist 26 times. An Ophthalmologist 13 times. My family doctor 7 times. I saw an Orthopedic doctor 2 times, and a Chiropractor 3 times. I had 14 Biofeedback sessions. Doctors prescribed steroids 6 times and ordered 11 Medical tests. How I wish that would have been the end of it, but there would be more tests and more doctor visits to come.

Shopping and going into stores became a nightmare. The florescent lights not only made my blurriness worse they gave me a pain behind my eyes. Within a few minutes of being exposed to florescent lights, I became distracted, confused and disorientated. After fifteen minutes I started to lose strength in my legs, and my coordination was off. For years I avoided going into certain stores because of their florescent lights.

My husband and I finally sold our condominium, but it took a long, drawn-out eighteen months. We moved into our ranch home in July. Our house was lovely. Even though my walk was unsteady and I used a cane, I was excited about mowing the lawn and planting flowers around the house. I met many of our neighbors and enjoyed decorating our new home. Life was good for the rest of the year.

CHAPTER 5

~ In Four Short Years - A Turning Point ~

The following fall I lost more leg control. That was the last time I would walk to the mailbox on my own two feet. I did not have enough strength in my legs, even with the use of a cane, to walk out to the mailbox and back. The thought of my being stuck inside the house forever was not an option for me. I purchased my first scooter. It was hard for me to believe that in four short years I went from walking normally, to using a cane for balance, and finally needing a scooter to get around outside.

Inside the house, I continued to use a cane to get around. My legs tired easily, so I had to make sure chairs were placed strategically everywhere around the house. The chairs allowed me to sit and rest whenever the need would arise. Using my cane and a doorknob I was able to get from inside the house into the attached garage and onto my scooter.

Buying a scooter was just the beginning of a life-changing year. I had been a smoker for many years. Within a few weeks time, I quit. It's not for the reason you might think. I couldn't walk around the house holding a cigarette in one hand, an ashtray in the other, and a cane in yet another hand. I didn't have three hands. Something had to go. I quit smoking.

The hardest decision I ever had to make was concerning my car. I owned a Ford Maverick with a 302 cu inch V8 engine. It was a 3 speed on the floor with a racers clutch. I loved that car. I did not want to stop driving, but my legs were too weak to safely work the pedals. I cried for weeks after I voluntarily stopped driving.

Operating a car equals freedom. It's the freedom to come and go as you wish. Now I understood the heartache older seniors go through when they have to give up their car keys. You can no longer jump into the car and take a quick trip to the grocery store. You have to ask other people to drive you around or run errands for you. It's definitely a life altering decision.

That was also the year I started a special diet for Multiple Sclerosis. When I was first diagnosed with MS, my Neurologist suggested I buy a book called The Multiple Sclerosis Diet

Book[6] written by Dr. Roy Laver Swank, MD., Ph D. and Barbara Brewer Dugan.

[6] Printed with permission The Swank MS Foundation
http://www.swankmsdiet.org/the-diet/
accessed 06/26/2017

In his book, Dr. Swank, who worked with MS patients for over 35 years, explained why his low-fat diet was good for those who have MS. His book lists foods to eat and foods to avoid. The section of low-fat recipes helped me create foods that I knew were acceptable on the diet. Dr. Swank's book and information about his diet can also be found for free online.

Around the time I was first diagnosed with MS, I learned of a famous actress who had MS. As my MS progressed, I kept track of how she was doing. We were on the same path for quite awhile. One night while watching a television special I noticed she was in a wheelchair and was shaking quite noticeably. It broke my heart to see her so frail. I wanted both of us to beat this terrible disease.

If you're reading this and you have Multiple Sclerosis, please take a look at Dr. Swank's book or go on the internet and do a search using the words "Swank Diet." His diet might possibly slow down the progress of your disease. It has for me. My husband and I are convinced that this diet has kept me from becoming bedridden.

As if having panic attacks and blurry vision wasn't enough, I developed a red rash on my face. It looked like I had small red bumps, like tiny pimples, across both of my cheeks. I made an appointment with a Dermatologist who told me I had rosacea, a form of adult acne. He advised me that the condition was common in adults and often times was incurable. The doctor prescribed a medication to make the rash go away.

Through pure dumb luck I discovered what was causing my red rash. One day while shopping for salt at the grocery store, I could not find the salt container with iodized salt. It was out of stock. I purchased a container of regular salt. Within days the red rash began to disappear. Something in my diet had changed. I became a food detective. After weeks of eliminating foods, I eventually discovered that the iodized salt was causing my rash. Although the regular salt did not cause a rash, I decided to buy organic sea salt from that day on.

The diagnosis of rosacea got me thinking. If a simple ingredient like iodized salt could affect my body, what other foods were working against me? I started paying attention to foods and how my body reacted or didn't react to them.

Desperate to be free of Multiple Sclerosis, I started a new treatment called Plasmapheresis.

A medical dictionary gives the following description. *"Plasma exchange, also known as Plasmapheresis, is a way to "clean" your <u>blood</u>. It works sort of like <u>kidney dialysis</u>. During the treatment, plasma -- the liquid part of your <u>blood</u> -- gets replaced with plasma from a donor or with a plasma substitute.*

People with some forms of <u>multiple sclerosis</u> use plasma exchange to manage sudden, severe attacks, sometimes called relapses or flare-ups. Their plasma could have certain proteins that are attacking their own body. When you take out the plasma, you get rid of those proteins, and symptoms may get better."[7]

[7]WebMD Medical Reference Reviewed by Jennifer Robinson, MD on August 07, 2016

http://www.webmd.com/multiple-sclerosis/plasma-exchange-ms   accessed 06/26/2017

Here is my explanation. The nurse used a needle and tubing to draw blood out of my left arm. The tubing carried my blood to a machine that took out my albumin and replaced it with new albumin. The tubing carried the new improved blood back to a needle inserted into my left ankle. The whole process took around an hour. When I returned home, a visiting nurse would arrive and give me a gamma globulin shot in my buttocks. The shot was to help my body fight off infection. I hoped and prayed that Plasmapheresis was going to heal me. I wanted my body to return to the way it was before MS. I wanted my old life back. Unfortunately, that is not what happened.

The Plasmapheresis treatments and shots continued for 13 weeks. I had completed half of the treatments when everything had to be stopped. A steroid I was taking made me sick. In addition to the blood purification process, I was taking the steroid Prednisone. The doctor stopped my treatments because I was experiencing bad side effects from the steroids. I was crushed. I desperately wanted the treatments to work. Plasmapheresis was supposed to cure me. From that moment on I decided to never, ever try an experimental drug or treatment again. The disappointment is too great for me if it doesn't work.

Years later my dad passed away. I felt his passing. He was in one city, and I was in another, but I knew the moment he passed. I was standing on the front porch saying goodbye to my husband. He was leaving to go up north. While my husband was talking, I thought of my dad. For a fleeting moment, I felt a light, upward feeling followed immediately by a sense of sadness. I knew my father had passed away. A telephone call a couple of hours later confirmed what I had felt.

My MS remained steady for the next several years. I bought a juicer and started drinking carrot juice. Several months into drinking the juice my face and hands started taking on an orange color. It didn't bother me because I was feeling stronger. My husband, however, wanted a doctor's opinion. The doctor said my orange color was not uncommon. He suggested I drink the juice every other day. Once I switched to every other day my orange face and orange palms went away.

Both my husband and I agree that the carrot juice was helping me. It's too bad we stopped. It took too much time and energy to do everything. Besides preparing the carrots, and juicing them, one of us had to clean the juicer. It all became a huge chore. Someday when someone invents a self-cleaning juicer, we'll try it again.

Until then I'll buy refrigerated carrot juice from the grocery store.

CHAPTER 6

From out of nowhere I had an urge to sing, so I bought a Karaoke machine. My husband was going to be away deer hunting, and I would be in the house all by myself. I could sing to my heart's content, and sing I did. My husband would go bow hunting every weekend starting the third week in September and continue until the second week of November. After bow season was over, gun season started in late November. Sometimes my husband was gone eleven days in a row.

Left alone I could sing my lungs out because no one was around to complain. At the end of the season, I made a CD of my best songs. It was a lot of fun. No matter how much fun it was, I believe God had a hand in my buying that karaoke machine. The singing strengthened my lungs. I believe all of that singing helped me fight Pneumonia the following Spring.

Four months later I came down with Pneumonia. To my surprise, I got it from my husband. He had been battling Bronchitis for months. The doctors at the hospital told me I had contracted Pneumonia from my husband. The virus that gave him Bronchitis gave me Pneumonia. When I first got sick, I thought I had the flu. For two days I was so sick, I slept 23 out of 24 hours. Worried about my health my husband called an ambulance to take me to the hospital. The hospital put me in a private room because my pneumonia was in the contagious stage. Visitors had to wear a mask when they came to see me. Just the reverse happened when I went for x-rays. Outside my room, I was the one who had to wear a mask.

The first night in the hospital I woke up in total darkness. The room was pitch-black. There were no sounds. None. I couldn't even hear my own breathing. I wondered if I was dead. I looked around for the bright light at the end of a tunnel. There was none. Slowly I started hearing noises as I shifted around in bed. I was alive. Thank you, God, I was alive.

Eight days later, after numerous chest x-rays, two different intravenous antibiotics, oxygen, and egg beaters for breakfast; I was transferred to a rehabilitation center. All my strength was gone.

I needed help getting out of bed and into a wheelchair. A bedpan was constantly by my side.

When I met the physical therapist for the first time, we immediately butted heads. Her goal was twofold. First, she wanted me to work on my hand and arm strength and dexterity. Second, she wanted me to work on my balance and walking. My one and only goal was to go to the bathroom by myself. After a long talk with the therapist, she understood my problem. I had a small amount of energy and if I did arm circles on a table, I wouldn't have enough stamina to do anything else. I desperately wanted to use what little energy I had to strengthen my legs. Two weeks of people wiping my buttocks after a bowel movement HAD to come to an end. The therapist understood, and for the next two weeks we worked on my leg strength. At the end of my stay, using a walker, I was able to slowly walk 30 feet without sitting down.

A month after first being admitted to the hospital I returned home. Waiting for me was a hospital bed. There were grab bars on the bed, next to the head area, that allowed me to pull myself up into a sitting position. The grab bars also provided something for me to hang on to while I transferred from the bed to a scooter. Having a scooter was a blessing. I was far too weak to wheel myself around in a wheelchair, and having my husband push me around in one was out of the question. Although it was my goal, I could not use the toilet in the bathroom. I had to use a toilet bench for months.

Don't know how I would have made it without my husband. He took over all the household tasks and chores. He cooked all our meals and washed our clothes. He emptied the toilet bench tray multiple times a day. His actions proved over and over again that he loved me, despite my disability. I thank God frequently for bringing this wonderful man into my life.

Finally, after nine long months, I was able to return the rented hospital bed. It felt wonderful getting into our bed beside my husband. Eventually, I was able to go to the bathroom and use the regular toilet. How I wish I could say everything was back to normal, but it wasn't. It took another year for my strength to return and for me to feel like I did before Pneumonia.

Two years later I developed Shingles. I had a four-inch red, pustule rash all across the small of my back. I also had a five-inch wide rash that completely encircled my right thigh. When I went to the doctor's office, I felt pretty good. The doctor offered to give me a shot that would speed up the healing process by a week. I thought "one week only? That's not a lot." I decided to skip the shot.

A couple of days later the pain started, and it was an intense pain. Anything that touched the shingles area caused great pain. Even the clothes I was wearing hurt like heck. I ended up wearing a long, mid-calf nightshirt. Unfortunately, the shingles affected my MS. A low-grade fever made my body weak and my legs wobbly. Once again I had to use the toilet bench. It's always nice to get your money's worth out of a product, but this was ridiculous.

The first week I slept in a recliner. I was too weak to get in and out of bed. My weakened immune system, due to MS, slowed down my healing time. It took over six months to completely get rid of Shingles.

At the beginning of 2012, I had a strong feeling something was going to happen in July. As the days grew closer, I started to get nervous. Was I going to get sick? Would my MS get worse? Would something horrible happen? I was on pins and needles the first day of July.

Mid-July my scooter stopped working, and when it broke down, it left me stranded outside. It was 9:00 pm and my scooter could not make it up the ramp into our house. My husband was out of town and would not be home for several hours. The whole situation left me frustrated. The front door was six feet away, but I could not get to it. Lucky for me a neighbor returned home a little after nine o'clock. He was kind enough to push me and my scooter up the ramp and into the house. The scooter had left me stranded several times before. I vowed it would never happen again. Within days I bought a new one. Thankfully my July mystery turned out to be the need for a new scooter.

The urgency I felt about the need to travel allowed me to fulfill part of my "Bucket List" early in life. If I had waited until I retired, I would have missed out on so much. Because I was young and worked for an airline, I was able to travel all over the world. In addition to the places I've already mentioned, I traveled to faraway places like Sidney, Australia; and Suva, Fiji. I traveled to Brussels, Belgium; Copenhagen, Denmark; London, England; Luxemburg City, Luxemburg; Dublin, Ireland; and Rome, Italy. Can't forget my travels to the Bahamas, and to multiple cities in Mexico and Canada. Last but not least, I traveled around our great country - from sea to shining sea.

Here is one of my favorite funny travel moments. While traveling on an around the world trip, I had won at an airline party, my girlfriend and I had to exchange our US dollars into the local currency. There were no Euros at that time. Each European country had their own currency. Several had an exchange rate of 3 to 1 while another one was 8 to 1. In Germany, we switched from dollars to Deutsche Marks. Switzerland had Francs. Greece had Drachmas. Thailand had Bahts. By the time we arrived in Hawaii, we had exchanged our currency five times. When we stopped at a McDonalds in Honolulu, my friend looked down at her US money and asked me what the exchange rate was!

Many times during my life I have had the feeling I was taking one step forward and two steps back. How I wish I didn't have MS. I want so badly to walk to the mailbox and back on my own two legs. An old English proverb from the 16th century says, "If wishes were horses, beggars would ride." Sometimes it's useless to wish for something that's out of your control.

An experimental treatment conducted at the University of Wisconsin-Madison caught my attention. The treatment would have made me "take back" my words of "*I'll never, ever try an experimental treatment again.*" The experiments were called cranial nerve non-invasive neuromodulation.

Here's a quick explanation of cranial nerve non-invasive neuromodulation. - *"The investigator's hypothesis is that electrical stimulation to the tongue that directly stimulates two cranial nerve nuclei (Trigeminal and Facial Nerve Nuclei), will excite neural impulses to the brainstem and cerebellum. The investigators call this cranial nerve non-invasive neuromodulation (CN-NINM). The activation of these structures induces neuroplasticity when combined with specific physical exercises, can reduce symptoms of advanced MS, targeting primarily postural stability (sitting and standing), upper extremity movement, and ability to perform self-transfers."*[8]

[8] ClinicalTrials.gov accessed 06/26/2017
https://clinicaltrials.gov/ct2/show/NCT02252666?term=cranial+
nerve+noninvasive+neuromodulation&rank=5

This is my understanding of what happened. A small electric device was used on the patient's tongue. The device used electrical stimulation of the tongue to essentially rewire the brain and bring about dramatic improvements in participants who had Multiple Sclerosis. The treatments consisted of twenty minutes of electrical stimulation of the tongue followed immediately with walking on a treadmill. Two weeks of these experimental treatments made an enormous difference for MS participants. All those who participated had improvements in their condition.

Sadly six months down the road, the improvements started to "drift away." It was said that patients might have to use the device for years to keep themselves in "normal" shape. My thoughts were, *"What's the problem with that?"* Here's a simple, non-invasive way a person with MS can improve their life. This might be a bad analogy but what's the difference between a woman taking her time to go to the Beauty Shop every six to eight weeks, or a woman taking her time to use the tongue stimulator every six months? If she has Multiple Sclerosis, they both would make her feel better.

CHAPTER 7

Update

Five years ago I ended my book at chapter 6. I agonized over whether or not I should release my book to the general public. I am not a professional writer, and I didn't know if anyone would be interested in what I had to say. Neighbors and friends urged me to share my experiences with others in the hopes that my book might help, or give hope to, someone else who might be dealing with Multiple Sclerosis.

~ Swank Diet ~

In chapter 5, I mentioned the Swank Diet. My husband and I are convinced that this diet helped delay the downward progression of my MS. Looking back over the years, it is hard to believe I have been on the Swank Diet for over thirty years.

When I was first diagnosed, I was not taking any drugs to treat my MS. Perhaps I should rephrase that statement. When I first started the Swank Diet my doctor told me there were no treatments for my kind of MS, Primary-Progressive Multiple Sclerosis (PPMS).

One of my biggest regrets is that I didn't start the diet sooner. I was in complete denial and had convinced myself that the disease would go away by itself. I have no good reason to tell you as to why I thought that, but I did. In my heart, I believed my healing was right around the corner. I refused to admit that I had a lifelong debilitating disease. That thinking stopped me from starting the Swank Diet right away.

What if I had started the diet sooner? Would I still be walking with a cane? Would I have better eyesight? Sadly I will never know the answers to my "what if's."

By the time I bought Dr. Swank's book and started the diet, I was already experiencing multiple symptoms. My understanding of what the book says, and these are <u>my</u> <u>words</u>, *the diet cannot give you back something you have lost, but it might slow down any new symptoms.* In my case, I believe this is true.

The first year on the diet was the hardest. I wish could tell you it was easy but it took dedication and determination on my part to stay on it. The first year you cannot eat any red meat.

No steak, no bacon, no bologna, and no hamburgers. That means no meat from a cow, a sheep, or a pig. (Sorry pork eaters but pork is considered red meat on this diet.) For the first 365 days, you will mostly eat chicken, turkey, or fish. There are some restrictions - so keep reading. Dark meat from chicken and turkey are permitted but limited. (Please see the book or the website for the particulars.)

In the beginning, I found the Swank Diet difficult to follow because I had to break my love affair with fast foods and fried foods. Many fast foods had one or two ingredients in them that were prohibited. I thought I would starve to death because so many of my favorite foods were off limits. The thought of having to fill up on fruits and vegetables made me shudder. No offense to Vegans, but I like meat.

The diet would be a challenge for me, but I had to make a life-changing decision. Either follow this diet exactly as instructed, or continue eating as usual and take the chance that I might get worse. If my MS continued on a downward trend, I could become bedridden. The thought of living my life in a bed scared me. Those thoughts pushed me to choose the diet.

When I first started, there were only a handful of items I could buy at our grocery store. Thank goodness for health food stores. I had to go there to buy my low-fat products. My husband and I had to become label readers. I began to hate the words partially hydrogenated oil. It was the primary source of artificial trans fat in processed foods. Years ago it was in everything. Well, practically everything. While reading the ingredient list on a product, my eye would go immediately to the middle of the list. That is where I usually found partially hydrogenated oil listed.

Happily, it looks like my trans fat reading days may be over. Companies will now have to comply with a new government regulation regarding triglycerides (partially hydrogenated oil) beginning June 18, 2018.

Many companies have already removed it from their products so more and more foods can be found on the shelves in your regular grocery store.

Regrettably, another prohibited food has begun to appear. Over the last ten years, the use of palm kernel oil has increased. Palm oil can be found in many food items. It is high in saturated fat and therefore not allowed on the Swank Diet. It looks like my ingredient list reading days are not over.

What else have I learned?

~ A Good Attitude ~

Throughout my life, different adults have urged me to "think positively." The minute they started speaking those words I heard "blah blah blah." How ironic it is that now I am asking you, the reader, to "think positively." I believe a good attitude has helped me over the years. Friends and neighbors who know me well, call me an optimist. Perhaps I was born that way. I don't know, but from young on I remember being a happy person. Whenever bad things happen, I try to find something good about the situation. More than once I have said to myself "it could be worse."

To help see the good side of life, I try not to get angry. Those are easy words to say; however, it's nearly impossible for someone to go through life without getting mad. We all get mad at the people in our lives like spouses, children, friends, and neighbors. Add traffic jams, barking dogs, bad bosses, computers glitches and a myriad of other things that can ruin your day, and we get mad.

Over the years I have learned that when I get mad, the only person who ends up getting hurt is me. Inadvertently my back and neck muscle tense up. My stomach tightens, and I end up with a stomachache. So the bottom line for me is, nothing good comes from holding on to anger.

~ Backaches ~

Years ago I used to do exercises to strengthen various muscles in my body. I'm embarrassed to say I stopped doing them. Most of the day I spend sitting in a chair or on a scooter. When I lean over to pull weeds or pick up a piece of paper off the floor, I can feel the pull on my back muscles. They start to tighten, and if I don't do something quickly to relax them, I'll pay for it later with back pain.

What do I do to head off the pain? It's not what you think. I have an aversion to taking pills - any kind of pills. To me, there is always a side effect of some kind. I have come up with my own way of relieving my simple back pain. I breathe. If you're rolling your eyes after reading that last statement, I understand. Everyone breathes but I came up with my own breathing exercises to help stop the pain before it gets started.

First, I part my lips and slowly draw in air through my teeth. You read that correctly, through my teeth. After breathing in, I exhale slowly through my mouth like I'm blowing out a candle. I do this two or three times in a row. Then I breathe normally for several minutes before I repeat the above two more times. I have to be careful not to do this too many times or for too long a period, because I don't want to hyperventilate.

Next, I rub my back muscles with the back of my hand. I do this for 20 seconds at a time or until my arm gets tired. I repeat this four or five times, spaced between my breathing exercises. An electric massager would work fine on my back but I find it faster and easier to use my hand.

The third thing I do is drink six to eight ounces of water. These three steps have helped me for over 10 years. They must be working because I have not taken any kind of pills or medication for pain, either from a doctor or purchased locally over the counter, for 13 years.

I repeat the breathing exercises and the back rubbing several times throughout the day. Please note that my exercises are a way for me to eliminate SIMPLE muscle pain. I am not a doctor, and I am not suggesting you try my exercises. I only wanted to share my experiences with you. Should you suffer back pain, please see your doctor.

~ Hyperventilate ~

In Chapter 7, I told you about my Biofeedback sessions and how it helped me control my breathing. Somewhere along the line, I went from slowing down my breathing to holding my breath whenever I face a stressful situation. When I hold my breath too long, I hyperventilate. The first time it happened, I ended up in an emergency room.

What happens when I hyperventilate? My body temperature begins to rise, and my neck and face become uncomfortably warm. Next, I become lightheaded. If I do not begin breathing regularly to stop it from going any further, I will begin to shiver uncontrollably. This is a critical time. It's imperative that my breathing return to normal or I will experience a full-blown panic attack.

Unable to break this horrible habit, I began singing an old song I remembered from childhood. Singing the song in my head, I breathe in and out with the words. The song forces me to breathe in a regular pattern. Does it help? Absolutely!

Here's the song.

(breathe in)   A-tisket
(breathe out) A-tasket
(breathe in)   A green and
(breathe out) Yellow basket
(breathe in)   I send a letter
(breathe out) To my mommy
(breathe in)   On the way
(breathe out)   I dropped it
(In)   I dropped it
(Out)   I dropped it

There's more to the song, but I think you get the idea. You may laugh at the song and my procedures, but it works for me.

CHAPTER 8

~ Rest ~

Whenever a new symptom develops, I try my best to rest and relax as much as possible. No stressful television shows. No loud or irritating music or sounds. The best place for me to rest is in bed, although the recliner comes in second. If possible, I try to rest a minimum of 30 to 40 minutes. Early on I learned that if I refuse to slow down and rest, my temporary new symptom will become permanent.

~ Shingles ~

In Chapter 6, I mentioned my very painful shingles rash. How sad it is that in 2017, years after my first bout of shingles, I suffered my 5th rash. Thankfully none of my reoccurring rashes were painful. Irritating, but not painful. It seems every time I experience a stressful situation; I get another shingles breakout. It looks like I'll have to work harder on my stress control techniques.

~ Vertigo ~

The first time I had vertigo, it scared me. All I did was turn my head, and I immediately felt light-headed and dizzy. I had to lie down on the couch, on my side and hope it would go away. Luckily I had laid down on my right side. Later I discovered that all my symptoms would get worse if I rolled over onto my left side or if I looked up and to my left. Eventually, the dizziness went away.

Afraid of another attack, I made an appointment to see my neurologist. He told me vertigo is common for those who have MS. That was not what I wanted to hear. I wanted it to be a one-time occurrence. I felt better when the doctor gave me a piece of paper with exercises I could do at home. I'm happy to say the exercises kept my vertigo under control. Unfortunately, it's a reoccurring problem that comes back whenever it wants. When it returns, I begin the exercises as quickly as possible.

Vertigo is nothing to take lightly, so I am hesitant to share my exercises with you. I would suggest you ask your doctor to recommend a physical therapist who can guide you through a few simple exercises or ask him to give you some exercises to try at home.

Other things I have learned.

~ Steroids ~

My body can no longer handle steroids without my having an adverse reaction. Even low doses affect me. Steroids helped me when I first took them, and they have helped <u>many</u> people with MS get over a bad situation. I won't say I will *never* take them again, but I will try to avoid them if possible.

~ Vitamin D ~

Blood tests have shown that I have a low level of vitamin D. Years ago I read somewhere that exposing your eyes to 20 minutes of sun was all you needed to get your minimum daily amount of vitamin D. I took that to heart and made sure I sat outside in the sun no matter what the season.

As far back as I can remember I have loved being in the sun. Sometimes I think I'm drawn to it. If it's a cloudy day, I feel no need to go outside. If the sun breaks through the clouds and shines brightly, I feel compelled to go outside. I often wonder if I've been deficient in vitamin D all my life and perhaps that's why I'm drawn to the sun.

Winter, Spring, Summer, and Fall I go outside when the sun is out. Neighbors are used to seeing me sitting on the porch even if it's ten degrees outside. One neighbor, in particular, likes to tease me saying it would be easier to just take a vitamin D pill.

I do not know if the amount of D I get helps me, but I do know it improves my mood. The warmth of the sun is relaxing even if it's mid-January and it's 20 degrees outside. If all the doctors in the world got together and told me there is absolutely no way I could get vitamin D during the month of January, I would continue to sit outside because it makes me feel good.

~ Barometric Pressure ~

My body is definitely affected by atmospheric pressure, more commonly known as barometric pressure. Whenever an approaching snowstorm or rainstorm is approximately 8 to 12 hours away, I can feel the barometric pressure changing because my body starts to feel different. For twenty minutes or so it becomes harder for me to breathe. I feel like an elephant is sitting on my chest. My entire body becomes heavy and it becomes more difficult to move. Thank goodness the pressure on my chest and the heaviness I feel is short lived. The symptoms usually last an hour or so before everything is back to normal.

Several people I know who have arthritis or have suffered a broken bone seem to know ahead of time when a storm is coming. Certain parts of

93

their bodies ache, and they know the weather is about to change.

Curious as to why approaching storms affected me, I started a list of the days and times when I felt bad. I called a local TV station and spoke with the meteorologist. She was kind enough to take the time to check her weather records against my list. We were both surprised to learn that I can feel the barometric pressure change 8 to 12 hours *before* a storm arrives in my neighborhood, AND I can feel it 6 to 8 hours *AFTER* it leaves. How unusual. I could feel the barometric pressure when it was on the rise AND when it was falling.

One fine summer day my rain predictions surprised everyone but me. My husband and I were going to go to a grandchild's baseball game. It started at 7:30 pm. It was a partly sunny day and the sun was peeking through the clouds when we arrived at the field at 7:00 pm. Several people sitting in the bleachers asked us why we had brought an umbrella. We told them we thought it was going to rain. Lo and behold, an hour later it began to sprinkle and then it rained.

It wasn't long before neighbors started asking me if I could feel a storm coming. They wanted to know if it was going to rain during their child's baseball game. I don't mean to brag, but I was right 90% of the time.

~ Listen to your body ~

Another thing I learned was to listen to my body. I thought I could eat every food that was approved on the Swank Diet, but I was wrong. I began to note my body's reaction to certain foods. Soon I discovered what foods caused a reaction and what foods did not affect me at all.

A perfect example is my body's reaction to beans. I love chili and I make a pretty good one. I knew ahead of time the lean hamburger I used in the chili would make me feel a little lethargic. It would also give me what I call brain fog and make my legs weak. Red meat also makes my body ache at night when I go to sleep. (More on that later) I accept all that knowing full well what is going to happen. That's why I eat chili when I know I'm going to stay home because I'm going to feel like a slug for a couple of hours.

One evening after eating chili I felt a whole new symptom. It was as if the back of my legs and everything nerve ending up and down my spine was on fire! What caused this new symptom? I had to find out.

When my husband went to the grocery store, he accidentally picked up a can of red beans instead of kidney beans. Uncertain as to whether or not the red beans were the culprit, I had the chili two nights later. Once again the nerves on the back of my legs and those along my spine were on fire. I cannot tell you why red beans hurt me and kidney beans don't. I can guarantee you that I will do everything I can to avoid red beans in the future.

~ Sleep ~

We all need sleep. Sometimes we crave it. Earlier in this book, I mentioned that red meat makes my body ache at night. Well, I found a natural way to calm the aches and pains. A slice of fresh pineapple or the juice from a quarter of a fresh lime squeezed into a glass of water helps me sleep more comfortably and soundly.

How did I learn that these two fruits would help me sleep? By accident. One day I had a craving for some pineapple but I did not want to go through the hassle and mess of coring one at home. I mentioned my dilemma to a neighbor who told me I could buy a fully cored pineapple at my local grocery store. I'm embarrassed to admit I did not know that. I'm probably the last person in the neighborhood who did not know you could buy a fresh cored pineapple.

Eagar for fresh pineapple, I ran to the store. Around 8:00 pm I cut off a slice about three-quarters of an inch thick and ate it. I slept for 5 1/2 hours straight! The only reason I woke up was because I had to go to the bathroom. Five and a half hours might not sound like a long time to the average person but for me, anything over three hours straight is okay in my book.

I learned about the benefits of using limes from a friend. She told me she added fresh lime juice to her water because it helped keep her body more alkaline than acidic. I had researched this information on the internet and I was ready to give it a try, especially after she told me it helped her sleep better.

Whenever I eat red meat or have a lot of wheat products for dinner, I cut off a quarter of a lime and squeeze the juice into a six-ounce glass of water. Nine out of ten times I sleep an average of five hours straight. That makes me feel more rested and energetic the next day.

CHAPTER 9

Gluten and High Fructose Sugar

~ Nosebleeds ~

Two or three times a week I would get a nosebleed in the morning. I had to know what was causing them so (here we go again). I started keeping a list of the foods I ate. Eventually, the list helped me pinpoint the food(s) that caused the nosebleeds.

My first breakthrough came when I figured out that one of the culprits was the noodles I had eaten with our spaghetti dinner. We like the long skinny spaghetti noodles that you draw into your mouth quickly with a loud slurping sound. They are made with semolina and durum flour. I love the noodles, but they are one of the reasons why I had a bloody nose. When we switched to egg noodles, the nosebleeds stopped.

Thinking I had solved the problem, I was surprised days later when I had another bloody nose. It had to be from something I had eaten for supper or for a late night snack because the nosebleed occurred the next morning. This time I narrowed it down to our store bought bread. I began buying different kinds of breads hoping one of them would not affect me. The nosebleeds continued. It was a sad day when I removed bread from our shopping list. With no bread to eat how was I going to make French Toast?

Things changed for me when my husband brought home a packet of six Kaiser buns. He bought them so he could make Sloppy Joe sandwiches. There was no way he was going to eat a Sloppy Joe sandwich in front of me! I had to have one. The next day I did not have a nosebleed. I was thrilled!

Kaiser buns contain semolina and durum flour so it baffles me to this day as to why I can eat those buns and not have a bloody nose the next morning. All I know is I can eat French Toast again!

To add more confusion to this whole gluten subject, I can make pancakes with unbleached white flour with no problems. White flour contains wheat. Wheat contains gluten. So why can I eat unbleached flour?

In the end, I discovered that if I eat regular bread (made without hydrogenated oil, of course) every 4 days, I have little reaction. Guess I'll have to wait for an expert to solve that and the Kaiser bun mystery.

~ Itchy Scalp~

As if nosebleeds weren't irritating enough, when I eat foods made with wheat I get an itchy scalp. The more gluten I ingest, the more my scalp itches. For thirty some years, I wrongly blamed the itching on a dry scalp.

~ Rosy Cheeks ~

In chapter eleven I mentioned a red rash that had developed on my cheeks due to iodine. The redness went away after I stopped buying iodized salt and switched to plain salt.

A few years ago a milder version of the red rash (more like a splotchy redness) began to appear on my cheeks. I call it rosy cheeks. To my surprise, the redness was caused by gluten! It happens whenever I eat a food made out of wheat. My cheeks go from rosy red to dark red it I eat wheat two days in a row. If I space it out to every four days I have no redness at all.

~ High Fructose Corn Sugar ~

High fructose corn syrup has been banned from my diet. I banned it. It's not that I don't love the sweet taste, but it makes me HYPER! After eating something with high fructose corn syrup in it, I do everything faster than normal. I talk faster and I become animated. Neighbors call it a "sugar buzz" and they know immediately when I've had some.

Thank goodness the cane sugar I cook with and put on my cereal doesn't affect me the same way.

~ One Last Word On The Swank Diet ~

In the beginning, I was a fanatic about sticking to the diet and not cheating. I said no to "just a nibble" and no to "just a bite." I drove family and friends crazy because I would not go off my diet "just this once."

Sometime in 2010 my willpower started breaking down. Thoughts like *"you only live once"* and *"I don't want to die without tasting that again"* began creeping into my thoughts. So far only three banned foods have broken my self-control. They are pizzeria Pizza, a locally grilled hamburger, and the best caramel pecan cinnamon buns in the world. I try to space them out to only one of the three each month. The rest of the time I stick to the diet.

Wish I could say the cheating hasn't affected me, but I believe it has. For over fifteen years I have used a walker inside the house and a scooter outside. In 2015, I began using a scooter occasionally in the house. A year later in 2016, I found I needed the scooter 50% of the time. It is obvious to me that my legs have grown weaker along with my hands and arms. The sad thing is I will never know why. Is it due to the debilitating effects of my disease, or is it because I've deviated from the Swank Diet?

If my condition takes a downward turn would I be willing to take a new drug called Ocrevus? On March 29, 2017, it was approved by the FDA to treat Relapsing Multiple Sclerosis AND Primary Progressive Multiple Sclerosis

(PPMS). This is the first drug ever to be approved for PPMS. Ocrevus is taken by IV infusion every six months. Will I run to try this new treatment? No. If the drug did not help me, I would be crushed. I will wait and let other people test it out first. Information on this drug can be found on the National Multiple Sclerosis Society website.[9]

[9]http://www.nationalmssociety.org/About-the-Society/News/FDA-Approves-Ocrevus
accessed 06/26/2017

~ Life's Blessings ~

What are the greatest things I have learned over the last twenty-five years? First on my list is the connection I have with my sister. It is a precious gift I cherish every day. Although far apart in miles we keep in touch regularly. My life would be less joyful and empty without her.

My stepchildren, their spouses, and my step grandchildren have each brought a bright spot to my life.

I am extremely fortunate to have the best neighbors and friends a person could ask for. My neighbors have come to my rescue time and time again. When I tipped my scooter over and was laying helplessly on the lawn, they ran to pick me up. Not only did they do it once, but twice. Hopefully, there won't be a third time. They have helped me in so many ways, it would take a page or two to list it all.

Three of my friends I have known longer than my husband. Although some of us have moved to different cities or different states, we have always managed to stay in touch. Emails and telephone calls keep us updated on the latest family news.

I thank God for all the good people in my life, especially my husband. As age and MS shrinks my world, it is comforting to know that my sister, or a close friend is just a telephone call or a text message away.

~ The End ~

www.ingramcontent.com/pod-product-compliance
Lightning Source LLC
Chambersburg PA
CBHW060418290526
45791CB00002B/800